Investing Wisely in Your Most Intimate Relationship

A Spiritual Life Growth Notebook for Singles

Andrea Hughes

authorHOUSE®

AuthorHouse™
1663 Liberty Drive
Bloomington, IN 47403
www.authorhouse.com
Phone: 1-800-839-8640

First published by AuthorHouse 2/16/2010

ISBN: 978-1-4490-4023-9 (sc)

Printed in the United States of America
Bloomington, Indiana

This book is printed on acid-free paper.

To my greatly supportive husband, John Edward Hughes, who continued on with home and business affairs while I was attending to completion of this book.

TABLE OF CONTENTS

ACKNOWLEDGEMENT

A special acknowledgement of the two editors of this manual, Cynthia Lewis and Dr. Gwendolyn Means for their commitment of time and helpful remarks and long time friend Sally King who did the final *average reader* comments which were so helpful. Young friend Cynthia has been a great resource and special support in my own spiritual growth.

FOREWORD

So many persons and ministries have played a significant role in directing my growth, some of whom will be mentioned in the text of this manual. However, I would like to highlight some of them here. First I acknowledge my mom, Beulah Leoda Edwards, who lovingly nurtured me and gave me a firm foundation in the Lord. For your reference, two ministries stand out among the numerous others that have influenced me. Campus Crusade for Christ, with its different urban ministry efforts, has led me to one of the most valuable tools of my prayer and reflection life, introduced by a humorous and generous lady presenter in a young women's seminar, *The Personal Daily Quiet Time,* also known as the P.D.Q.T. Then there is the Radio Bible Class which in addition to its many other ministries and publications, offers a monthly *Our Daily Bread* booklet available FREE from RBC Ministries. These two resources can be used beautifully together, as will be shown in this manual. Then there is the work written by Anne Ortlund, *The Disciplines of the Beautiful Woman,* one of the best tools for developing a rich spiritual life for *busy* women that I have ever had the great pleasure to stumble upon. Outstanding and recommended by a younger, serious Christian friend is Richard Foster's classic *Celebration of Discipline: The Path to Spiritual Growth* revised and expanded. This is another major contemplative tool that helped me round out and more fully understand who I was as a Christian and more about who Jesus is. What's so great about these last two books is that neither is lengthy. You will more than likely want to have your own personal copy of these two resources for marking and revisiting.

During the course of this notebook I will not only be recommending spiritual disciplines but books that helped me carry them out. A list of recommended books is included both in the back of Richard Foster's book and this one, which should also prove helpful to *your* spiritual growth and intimacy.

This book is for those who feel like they are being tainted by or swept up in the fast current of the secular world, who want to be *loved* and *accepted* and who want to *love purely*, who want to *slow it down*, and *grow deeper* in their spiritual walk, and who want to leave an impact on the world for His Majesty, and possibly guide others behind them into this life. I hope it is a special treat.

Chapter One - How This Book Came About

This book came about through my desire to see more growth and richness in my spirituality and relationship with the Lord Jesus and to share it with others. As a young person growing up in a devout Christian home around a mom who practiced as much as she preached, I witnessed a life of piety that many of my generation and the ones behind me did not have the blessing of sharing. My sisters and brother discovered this too, as we opened our home-made double-decker sandwiches, thickly stuffed with chicken, tuna or whatever Mom could find, and a handwritten Bible verse on perfectly cut notebook paper tucked right in between the 3 bread layers. Our elementary school lunch mates always wanted to know what these verses said. They were unusual "fortune cookies" or buried treasure to them. The same thing happened with "care" packages sent to me in college and far away in my first job. In my mother, I witnessed a woman who actually "prayed without ceasing". I used to wonder, as did the grandkids in future years, to whom Mom was talking and listening. She would answer us all with a smile, "the Lord". We saw her rising at 5:00 a.m. in the morning to be with her Bible, taking copious notes, writing in the margins with a hymnal near by and thought her habit was intriguing. Then there were the journals in which she kept life-notes and the prayer meetings she hosted at our house. I also sometimes attended such meetings at the homes of others, with her and my Dad. Sometimes they took us to Bible studies at a church whose religion we didn't even belong to, but which was led by an outstanding teacher. This was a great shepherd, teacher of preachers, who handed out one page of outlined typed notes each time. He always started out the packed, small church Bible study with worship and the song: "None but the righteous (repeated 3 times), shall see God", sung in the old Black Southern worship style.

It was these and more such traditions that I found peculiar to our family that have helped me in my spiritual growth and foundation. They also kept me from some dangerous choices. My interest was peaked as to how people like my mom, the spiritual elders, and great saints became their confident, simple living, seemingly unruffled, at peace, trusting-God selves.

How did such a group of real people of faith whom I have consistently been drawn to over the years, do this? All of them seemed to have busy lives, involved with activities either in the neighborhood or community and who spent quality time raising their children or with relatives and friends. They still maintained life styles that included quality time with God, not allowing this time to be choked out by other activities. I saw and have experienced people who lived a life walking in and with the Holy Spirit, in everyday, humble (and sometimes classy) neighborhood surroundings. It was attractive. Some of their secrets I discovered from watching my mother and others with similar life habits, hanging around these people who seemed to me to be giants of the faith, and reading rich Christian books.

As a person living in an urban environment with a "Martha" active personality, I have found it more and more difficult to live the type of life which these afore mentioned busy but focused listeners-to-the-Spirit pursued. Moreover, I have found more and more Christians who do not even know how to live a life of peace, not assimilating into the mainstream of secular society norms. This spiritual growth notebook is dedicated to all those in the quest of "the holy," but living in the mundane, busy, rat-race world. I'll try to clearly share with you - who want to be more focused in growth, enjoy living your faith more, and grow up more quickly in the most intimate of relationships - a few of the practices I found which helped me along the way as a teenager, a young adult, a single adult and as a married person.

This notebook is divided into several sections each having pages of blank sheets to try out some of the disciplines and practices I have found helpful. Richard Foster mentions 12 disciplines in his classic book, dividing them into 3 types: *The Inward*: meditation, prayer, fasting, and study; *The Outward*: simplicity, solitude, submission, service; and *Corporate*: confession, worship, guidance, and celebration.[1] Every one of them is so important to your spiritual growth. However, the content, understanding and life Foster brings to these disciplines are what are so key to "real" spiritual growth. Not a book to be read quickly, his book will fill in the details of what you don't find on the spiritual disciplines here. I return to it and other similar works time and time again.

You will be introduced to a format and style to help you remember and use the disciplines found in this notebook. Anne Ortlund introduced this notebook style to me through her short study book – *The Disciplines of the Beautiful Woman*. I have had the privilege of facilitating several groups of many women who wanted to get a grip on their hectic lives to add more quality and depth. Utilizing this book for those study groups was of great benefit to the spiritual growth of all of us. Through their sharing of other notebook

---

1.   p. v. Contents. Richard J. Foster. *Celebration of Discipline*. Revised and Expanded edition.

formats and other sharings from companions along the way, a notebook was developed that has worked for me.

The notebook and disciplines' emphasis have been altered as my life and my emphasis on various disciplines have ebbed and flowed depending on what was occurring in my life. You are urged to adapt and find what is most comfortable for you. Keep in mind that the Old Testament Jews were not (for the most part) assimilated or marginalized, into the pagan cultures that captured them or elsewhere they were dispersed. It is notable that one of the main reasons for this was their observance of the Law, *torah* (instruction), and by their *continued observance of the pattern of life* maintained in Palestine, their homeland. This is according to H.L. Ellison in his article in the International Bible Commentary edited by F.F. Bruce.[2] Could this help explain why you now cannot tell us Christians from the secular world today? Is it because we lack the observance of the disciplines and pattern of life the early church practiced and instead conform to the secular (and pagan) world around us?

This is my experience. It worked well for me. However each personality type, by seeking God's face, will find the best way to draw closer to Christ. May you be mightily blessed by the Holy Spirit in this venture to recapture or maintain a deeper observance of the life Christ lived and come into all that He promised of the "abundant life"!

"...until we all reach unity in the faith and in the knowledge of the Son of God and become mature, attaining to the whole measure of the fullness of Christ. Then we will no longer be infants, tossed back and forth by the waves, and blown here and there by every wind of teaching and by the cunning and craftiness of men in their deceitful scheming. Instead, speaking the truth in love, we will in all things grow up into him who is the Head, that is, Christ." Ephesians 4:13-15 (New International Version of the Bible -NIV) (Emphasis added.)

---

2.   p. 1053. F. F. Bruce, General Editor. H.L. Ellison, article editor, *The International Bible Commentary.*

Chapter Two - How To Use This Book

You can use this book as is for a trial period. After you read through it once, you are encouraged to buy a 3-ring notebook, 8 1/2 by 11, take the spine off this book, pull the pages, and get 3 holes punched in them to start your own Growth Notebook. You may prefer to photocopy the sections for your notebook rather than take the book apart or to purchase two books, one to disassemble and one to stay intact. Just remember this is a *spiritual growth* workbook to help you move forward, grow deeper and *see* your progress. Each year you may want to add more to it and change its sections. 8 1/2 by 11 sized paper is always available, affordable and often on sale, which is why, I chose this format. Feel free to copy the section breaks and pages and reduce them in size for fitting a smaller 6-hole *day-timer* notebook available at office supply and some "dollar" stores. You can also keep bookmarkers, tracts, prayer cards, and your *Through the Bible* schedule in the pockets of your personally developed notebook. Look for the notebooks that have the plastic cover you can slip an identifying cover page in and inside pockets to slip the items I listed above and more. Index tabs placed on the side of the beginning page of each section and labeled will help you find the sections faster. You can use tab-size Post-its and label them to get the same ease of location.

If you find, after going through this manual, that all this discipline material lacks luster, is dry, or really not appealing to you at all right now, you may want to read the two small brief pamphlets produced by Campus Crusade for Life: *The Four Spiritual Laws* and *Have You Made the Wonderful Discovery of the Spirit-filled Life?* Order information is in the Appendix Section. Many churches and ministries give them away free.

Feel free to write or call in about customizing your notebook:

By mail: Abundantly Living Services,
1226 Jackson St. NE, Wash. D.C. 20017

By phone: Voice: 202-269-3449

By internet: Email: princessayh@hotmail.com
Website: www.abundantlylivingserv.com

Enjoy this period of trying on new growth outfits as you invest even more wisely in your most intimate relationship.

"Draw near to God, and He will draw near to you." James 4:8 (New American Bible - NAB)

Chapter Three - How This Book Is Organized

To see great strides in this most important relationship there must be discipline and intentionality.

Section One – Intentional Calendars. Because time so easily slips away, it is very helpful to keep track of what you are doing in an intentional way. Using both a small at-a-glance calendar and a large monthly calendar help to avoid double booking and overbooking. Add calendars of your choice size and appeal in this section. Make sure they are large enough to write important activities you don't want to miss.

Section Two – Accountability Partner/Group. This is an important discipline to *everyone* growing in this intimate relationship. God is spirit. We love him and are trying to draw nearer by knowing his son Jesus. However, we need some human support, community, and guidance. This is where small groups, mentors, spiritual directors/ companions, accountably partners come in.

Section Three – Goals. Goals are so important in helping us say "yes" to some activities and calls on our lives and "no" to others that take us away from where we really want to go, be and value most. See the chapter "Saying Yes and Saying No" by M. Shawn Copeland in Dorothy Bass's *Practicing Our Faith* and the first sections of Steven Covey's *Seven Habits of Highly Successful People* for some additional help here. Dividing goals into small chunks as outlined in this section has helped immensely in realizing the long-term and short-term plans for life. The last part of these chunks, "Month Goals," is a special treat: Great, Delightful/Uplifting Experiences You Had This Month. This is a praise and thank you-oriented, "memorable moment" section to cheer you up and to remind you that God loves you and is faithful. It helps a lot in disappointing or dreary times. Maintaining a book of these jewels has proven to me to be very uplifting.

Section Four – A Personal Devotion "Lover's" Time. This time is different from your Bible study and your contemplation time, even though some of us use it as a short meditation time. A format is given to assist with employing this special intimate spiritual growth practice. The splendor of a lengthier time is also introduced.

Section Five – Bible Study and Scripture Memorization. Here is emphasized knowing more *about* the One who is the focus of this growing intimate relationship, how He operates, what is required to best relate, and His expectations. The sheets "Verses I Am Learning" are an addition to help in keeping track of selected verses you will want to learn over a period of time for a variety of reasons. You may choose to note the subject and scripture sources here or just the subject.

Section Six – Sermon Notes. These notes can be from Sunday sermons, along with those obtained while listening to a radio, TV or Internet program and tucked here. They can also be written on other notepaper and stapled here when your notebook is not available.

Section Seven – Growth Aides: Books, Tapes, CD's, and Audio-Visuals list. Using a variety of sources for your spiritual growth can help you delve into the riches of the King and Kingdom in a different way. Sometimes you may want to look back at a resource or recommend it to someone. Listing them monthly helps one remember and realize some of the progress you are making and the direction in which you are being led.

The Appendix contains source information that hopefully will prove more than helpful on your journey.

Spiritual Life Growth Notebook Owner's Page

This notebook belongs to:

Name _____

Address _____

                                Street   apt. #

_____

                             City   State   Zip

Best phone number for reaching me _____

My Accountability Partner/Group Name:

_____

Prayer partner, spiritual director, mentor, support group, Cursillo group reunion. These may change over the years or stay the same for many years.

Regular Meeting Time

_____

Being accountable to someone or to a group is so helpful in objectively seeing our weak areas, discerning situations, prayer support on concerns, rejoicing about areas of growth and sharing of testimonies and many other aspects shared one on one or in small groups that cannot be shared with large ones. Jesus also had his small groups of intimates.

"For none of us lives to himself alone and none of us dies to himself alone." Romans 14:7 (NIV)

Section One

Intentional Calendars

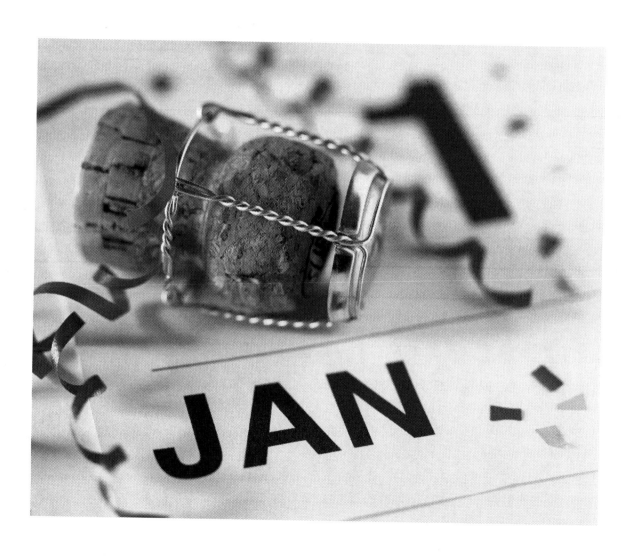

Current year Calendar here

Following year Calendar here

SECTION TWO
Accountability Partner/Group

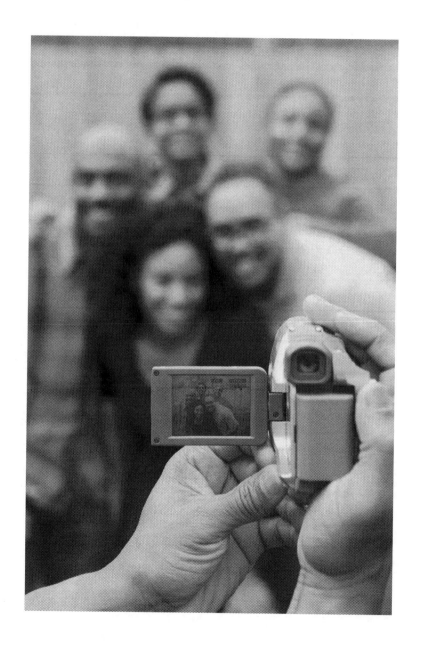

Dates I meet with my Accountability Partner/Group This Year

Circle below:

(Small calendar here)

""Therefore, confess your sins to one another and pray for one another, that you may be healed. The fervent prayer of a righteous person is very powerful." James 5:16 (NAB)

See Chuck Swindoll's *Living Beyond A Life of Mediocrity, p.291* for more on this topic and Richard Foster's chapter on accountability entitled "Guidance" in *The Celebration of Discipline.*

SECTION THREE
Goals

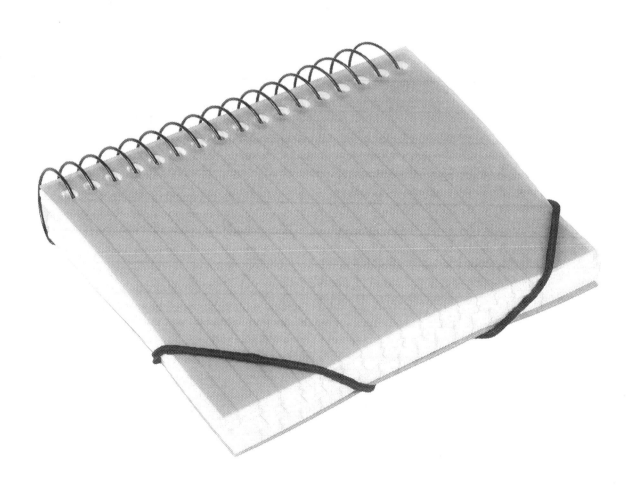

Goals

Life Goals – What you want to do with your life. Where do you want to be, and what do you want to have done before you die or are called in for your eternal reward, which, of course, could be tomorrow?

Anne Ortlund recommends **"3 Priority Areas"** which helped me frame the answer to these questions for a more spiritual focus:

1.   Knowledge of God, becoming more like Jesus
2.   Care for those of the Kingdom of God
3.   Care for those of the world

You may want to write you goals in list format. However, paragraph form works just as well. Do set some time aside to ponder these. You may want to rewrite them after reading through Ortland's *Disciplines*, Stephen Covey's *7 Habits of Highly Effective People,* Patrick Klingaman's *Finding Rest When the Work Is Never Done* or Kerry and Chris Shook's *One Month to Live: Thirty Days to A No-Regrets Life.*

Yearly Goals - Yearly goals should flow from your life goals. Identifying key roles and relationships you want to impact is very helpful here. I found about 10 that were plugged into those 3 Priority Areas was enough for me. These helped me live out the Life Goals and keep them in manageable chunks. Klingaman's chapter "Schedule Your Life with Purpose," based on Covey's first few chapters in *Seven Habits of Highly Effective People,* really proves beneficial here.

Monthly Goals – Monthly goals help you to keep close tabs on whether you really are accomplishing what you set out to do during the year toward your Life Goals. Who wants to reach the end of their life and find they have not done half of what they wanted to do?

Emilie Barnes' *My Daily Planner* book was very helpful here. She introduced me to a consistent examination of each month to check on:

> ➢ what was actually accomplished

> ➢ what prayers were answered

> ➢ uplifting experiences (which I was already recording in a "Book of Pearls" I had begun in my young adult years to help me become more grateful and cheer me up when I've felt "blue" and down or unloved)

> ➢ how my Bible study was going and my broader reading of materials to help me become well rounded and informed both of Kingdom affairs and the larger world where we Christians serve as leaven. I enlarged the resource materials to embrace not only books and print materials but also other media as well.

Weekly Plan to Attain Goals - As a career woman and later as a wife, I found that having a couple of these planner sheets has been tremendously helpful in focusing on my three priority areas. Breaking them down into smaller manageable tasks gave me a chance to gain a sense of accomplishment. Seeing myself make gains in what I wanted to do with my life has been uplifting. Making sure the weeks of the month didn't slip by without me getting any of my monthly goals taken care of, plus avoiding being blown away at the end of the year when I found there were no major dents in accomplishing my *year* and *life goals*, were well worth all this planning.

Linda Dillow's *Priority Planner Notebook* has been tremendously helpful with my home life planning. I still use her planner sheets. Having the week broken down into the focus areas she suggested with appropriate verses of scripture accompanying each area has been very useful. These areas are entitled: the LORD, HUSBAND (I substituted Friends and Relatives while single) CHILDREN (I substituted Disciples), HOME, YOURSELF (I loved this section. So thoughtful. Too many of us, especially women, forget to take care of ourselves when God orders us to love ourselves first before we can love our neighbor. Praise God!), and OUTSIDE THE HOME. Linda even had a Menu and Shopping List section for each week. This proved a little bit too much planning for me most of the time. What keeps this manageable and the user's life less hectic was Linda's orders to only have one task under each heading. This keeps the sence of being overwhelmed down and the sense of accomplishment up.

You can find great *business* planner sheets in most office supply stores and sometimes in the stationary section of other stores, even the "dollar" store. Slip them right in your notebook. You may have to enlarge them or find a suitable way to fit them with the rest of your growth notebook or carry them separately electronically like those using Black Berrys and various palm schedulers do. Just make sure you check your monthly calendar and goals to assure you are keeping these goals in mind and not over-booking yourself.

A large, monthly wall calendar (many come in the mail, are given out at church or are available in most gift, office supply and paper goods stores), which fits in your notebook to write specific activities and appointments on, helps you avoid double booking. Many have said that utilizing a large wall or refrigerator calendar for all the family to see and take note of, helps parents, spouses, and children plan or coordinate activities as a united group.

"Plans fail for the lack of good counsel, but with many advisers, they succeed." Proverbs. 22:29 (NIV)

My Life Goals

1. _____
   _____

2. _____
   _____

3. _____
   _____

4. _____
   _____

5. _____
   _____

6. _____
   _____

*"Praise the Lord. Blessed is the man who fears the Lord, who finds great delight in His commandments. His children will be mighty in the land; the generation of the upright will be blessed. Wealth and riches will be in his house, and his righteousness **endures forever.**"*
Psalms 112:1-3 (NIV)

My Goals for the Year 20

<u>Priority Area:</u>

1. _____
2. _____
3. _____
4. _____
5. _____
6. _____
7. _____
8. _____
9. _____
10. _____

"I will instruct you and teach you in the way you should go; I will counsel you and watch over you." Psalms 32:8 (NIV)

Goals for the Month of _____ Year <u>20</u>_____

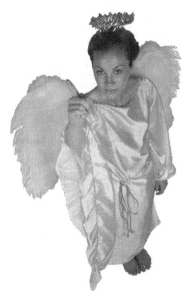

Don't forget to check your goals for the year and life goals!

Goals: _____

_____

_____

_____

Great Things that Happened This Month

_____

_____

_____

_____

"Whatever your task, work heartily, as serving the Lord and not men, knowing that from the Lord you will receive the inheritance as your reward; you are serving the Lord Christ."
Colossians 3:23-24 (Revised Standard Version of the Bible)

Section Four
Personal Devotions

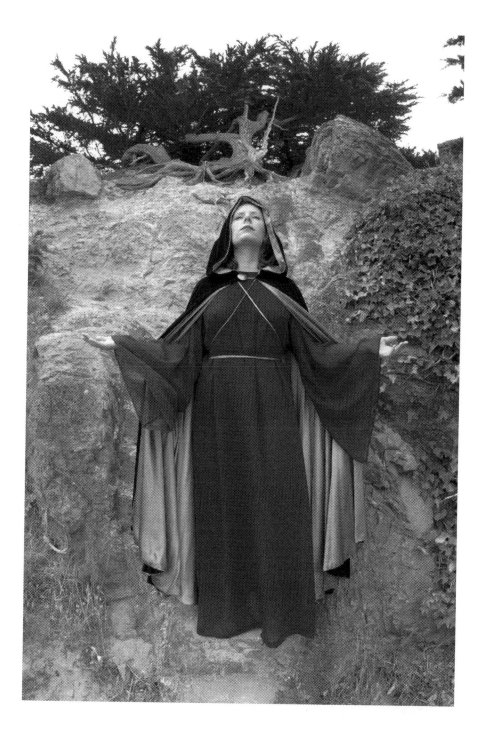

A Personal Daily Quiet Time (P.D.Q.T.)

Personal devotions is The Lover's Time for God to speak to our hearts and love us as we are still before Him in worship, praise, meditation on scripture. This is different from your Bible study. You get to know the son Jesus personally in order to become more like Him and love Him more. You receive guidance for the day, inspiration for the heart and have Him control or influence your life on a daily basis. In a Bible study you learn more *about* the father God and the son Jesus – facts, dates, places, how He works etc. by using guides such as concordances, maps and dictionaries.

Anne Ortlund reconfirmed my belief in practicing a Daily Quiet Time with the Lord. Only a short time is needed. **For energy and enlightenment, it's an especially great way to start a day.** She also recommends taking longer chunks of time for at-home and away retreats. Other such extended quiet times could include: days of reflection and seasonal "Quiet Days" during Advent and Lent (preparation for Easter). Do explore them. Try retreat houses and groups that offer spiritual growth opportunities. These I have found so valuable to my own spiritual growth and sense of being loved and the growth of those with whom I have shared these practices. **More about these below.**

A sample of a P.D.Q.T. format from a Campus Crusade seminar mentioned earlier in this book follows. This structure has proven very helpful in developing and keeping a special time with our Lord. The use of this format can not only help your written prayer blossom as mine did, but moreover your meditations may grow more in insight and application to your life. This format is highly recommended! Feel free to contact me for the complete outline and discussion.

You may wonder: *What do I need for an effective P.D.Q.T.?* Here are some helpful suggestions from the lady who passed it on to me in the Harambee class:

    A.   Proper rest and nutrition

    B.   Definite time and place free from all distractions

    C.   Good study Bible (with Concordance, cross referencing), a dictionary

    D.   Prayer before, during and after PDQT

1. Confess any unknown sins (before PDQT) that might hinder this time

2. Be still

3. Have a spirit of expectancy

4. Record daily in a journal how God spoke to you.

You may also find it hard to have a P.D.Q.T. Here are some roadblocks she suggests you will need to overcome:

A. Unconfessed sin

B. Haven't truly trusted Jesus as my personal savior – not a believer

C. I don't want to record it

D. Disorganization

E. Too lazy

F. No time

G. I'm tired

H. I don't know how

Do press on and remember her wise counsel:

"*When I wisely invest in God's word and apply it to my life and share it with others, then God will bless.*

GOD SAID IT!　　　**I BELIEVE IT!**　　　**THAT SETTLES IT!**"

It is suggested you use a separate tablet for your devotions. Use the following P.D.Q.T. page format when you are away from your regular tablet or notebook. Transfer (staple or paste) these back-up pages to your regular P.D.Q.T. notebook when it is available again.

The Radio Bible Class *Our Daily Bread booklet*, which comes out monthly, or utilizing a daily readings devotional such as the *Upper Room* booklet, *The Word Among Us* or Oswald Chambers' *My Utmost for His Highest,* are all great tools for use here. You can request the *Our Daily Bread* booklets **free** from: Radio Bible Class, Grand Rapids, Michigan 49555-0001. Donations are accepted of course. Their pamphlet: "Time with God" gives some explanation and "how-to tips". There are other such helpful pamphlets out there. For example, The Navigators' "How to Have a Quiet Time" from Navpress is one that you may want to check also.

My Personal Daily Quiet Time for

Time_____   Date_____

A.   Scripture verse or verses God impressed upon me:

     1. _____

     2. _____

B.   **Key Insights, Write Out** the impression God has given you through the verses you just read.

_____

_____

_____

C.   Personal Application: How can I apply God's impressions to m*y life?*

_____

_____

_____

D.   Personal Prayer: Write out.

_____

_____

_____

If God has just spoken to you about a certain area in your life that you need to yield to Him or have just yielded, **thank Him for it.** (Ephesians 5:20) **Be creative in your prayer response.** Sing a song or one of the Psalms to the Lord in praise.

E. Key Verse: Ask the Lord to help you memorize it. You might memorize the verse or verses you used for your P.D.Q.T.

_____

_____

_____

F. Optional: You might give your P.D.Q.T. a title Example: Full Life in Christ from St. John 10:10. (I have found this a very useful habit.)

"Those who look to Him are radiant; their faces are never covered with shame."
"Taste and see that the Lord is good, blessed is the man who takes refuge in Him." Psalm 34:3, 8 (NIV)
"The Lord appeared to us in the past, saying: **"I have loved you with an everlasting love; I have drawn you with loving-kindness."** *"*Jeremiah 31:3 (NIV) (Emphasis added)

Longer Quiet Times

Mini-retreats or one-hour retreats are great ways to celebrate "The Lovers times" too. Singing and dancing before the Lord during these times alone with Him are quite appropriate and lots of fun, besides being enriching. Do have a hymnal or 2 for these times. Indulge in praise and worship song and dance. Create your own – a new song. You might also try sitting, being with God, doing nothing. Use a place as quiet and free of distraction as you can find, where you can consider or contemplate and enjoy His glory and wonder, especially in nature. Whispering a single prayer word or phrase like "love" or "God loves me," "Jesus loves me," or one of the many names God has given Himself – El Shaddai -*God Almighty, The All Sufficient One*, Adonais – *My Great God*, Jehovah Rapha – *The Lord Who Heals*, Jehovah Jireh –*The Lord Will Provide* is helpful to focus yourself and quiet your mind.

Taking the time for these longer meditations, contemplation, is one of the best things you can do for your self, your love life, your temple maintenance. I have found that not only am I rejuvenated and refreshed but often I gather great insight and new ideas about matters that have been on my mind. Sometimes it's just a sense of being loved, like a great date with someone who really wants to be with you to show you lovely things like an exquisite sunset, a rolling lawn or yard covered with the natural wonder of fire flies, the quiet beauty of a simple sunrise with birds chirping as the earth awakens, fields of waving corn or wild flowers, night skies covered with stars, even a falling star! These kinds of things you don't notice when you are running around or busy, busy, busy with whatever. You really don't have to do anything, say anything or learn anything. Just be. Relax and be in His company, the company of the one who loves you most.

Only when you step away, take off and allow your mind to take a rest, allow your self to do nothing but being in God, the Divine's presence, do you get the glimpses of His special majesty and wonder and the sense that you are being specially treated because you took time on the planet to sit, sit and just be, be with Him. Being still. Being still and knowing more of this God. Enjoy!

A good way to preserve these times in order to reflect on them again is keeping a journal. Journaling, different from keeping a *daily* diary, is a great relaxation, relief tool, that almost everyone who does it reports only favorable outcomes. Not only can you use it as a preserver of treasured memories but it can be used also as a therapy - a teacher, reminder, and even vehicle for venting.

Check your Christian publishers, especially among the Catholic publishing houses, for pamphlets on how these delightful experiences can become part of your life. See also a list of resources at the back of this manual, which it is hoped will prove helpful.

"Be still and know that I am God." Psalms 46:10 (NIV)

" In repentance and rest is your salvation, in quietness and trust is your strength, but you would have none of it." Isaiah 30:15 (NIV)

"People and things come and go. But the spiritual satisfaction Christ offers sustains us in this world and will endure into eternity." Dennis Fisher. *Our Daily Bread* booklet, December 4, 2008

SECTION FIVE

Bible Study & Scripture Memorization

Bible Study

Getting to know God for yourself, including how God interacts with man, and His defining traits, is what this is about. This is what saved a few people from the famous Jim Jones cult communal suicide many years back. Studying to know how God operates with man has kept me from following some preaching and teaching that only learned ears would know was false teaching. This discipline of studying specific books of the Bible, reading through the Bible in its *entirety*, and *using good reference books such as*: Bible handbooks, Bible commentaries, various Bible translations, Bible atlases and concordances (Bible indexes), has definitely helped me stay with the truth rather than the latest whim of fast, smooth-talking teachers and preachers. I find there is so much "feel-good" teaching out there now that I have to go back and check the Holy Book, meditate, and ask other serious Bible studiers questions to make sure I'm hearing real truth.

Reading through the Bible each year, whether in its entirety or by studying the Old Testament one year and the New Testament the next year, keeps the knowledge of the magnitude of God – His goodness, His mercy, His faithfulness and His great love for us, fresh and fosters growth. You will find you are also better able to help others who are searching for truth.

Each year in reading through the Bible I find something I have not seen before. After all, the Lord Jesus did say that this is the *living word*. "It is the spirit that gives life; the flesh profits nothing. The words that I have spoken to you are spirit and life." John 6:64.

A number of through the Bible in a year type books, tracts and pamphlets are available. American Tract Society of Garland, Texas, www.atstracts.org, 1-800-54-TRACT, carries them by the package and for a Catholic version covering the Bible and the Catholic Catechism in a year try: CHResources of Zanesville, Ohio at www.chnetwork.org and 740-450-1179 or your Christian book stores. See Tim LaHaye's *How to Study the Bible for Yourself* for some practical ways and formats to approaching Bible study. Following is a sample study format.

"All Scripture is God-breathed and is useful for teaching, rebuking, correcting and training in righteousness, so that the man of God may be thoroughly equipped for every good work." I Tim. 3:16-17 (NIV)

Bible Study Sheet

Book_____   Date_____

Chapter/s_____

Theme _____
_____

Lessons for you about God. What is he saying to you? _____
_____
_____
_____
_____
_____
_____
_____
_____
_____
_____
_____
_____

"Indeed, the word of God is living and effective, sharper than any two-edged sword, penetrating even between soul and spirit, joints and marrow, and able to discern reflections and thoughts of the heart." Hebrews 4:12 (NAB)
"I have hidden your word in my heart that I might not sin against you." Psalm 119:11 (NIV)

Scripture Memorization

Memorizing scripture, "hiding the word in our hearts," is another important discipline that all Christians of this era do well to continue. With persecution against Christianity growing more and more and false doctrine increasing, to know the Word is even more important in staying on the straight and narrow. Also, you will enjoy being able to pull up important verses for yourself any time. Carrying a small pack of verses around in my pocket or purse has been a habit from teenage years. It helps keep you sharp mentally and morally and it allows you to help others when they need a specific encouragement. Campus Crusade and other ministries offer helpful memorization methods.

"Let the Word of Christ dwell in you richly..." Colossians 3:16a (New American Bible NAB)

"But if you make yourselves at home with me and my words are at home in you, you can be sure that whatever you ask will be listened to and acted upon." John 15:9 (The Message Bible)

Verses I Am Learning 20____

*Date*_____

*Subject:*_____

Verses' source- Name of books, chapters, verses _____

*Date*_____

*Subject:*_____

Verses' source _____

*Date*_____

*Subject:*_____

Verses' source _____

*Date*_____

*Subject:*_____

Verses' source _____

*Date*_____

*Subject:*_____

Verses' source _____

*Date*_____

*Subject:*_____

Verses' source _____

"And don't for a minute let this Book of The Revelation be out of mind. Ponder and meditate on it day and night, making sure you practice everything written in it. Then you'll get where you're going; then you'll succeed." Joshua 1:8 (The Message translation of the Bible)

SECTION SIX
Sermon Notes

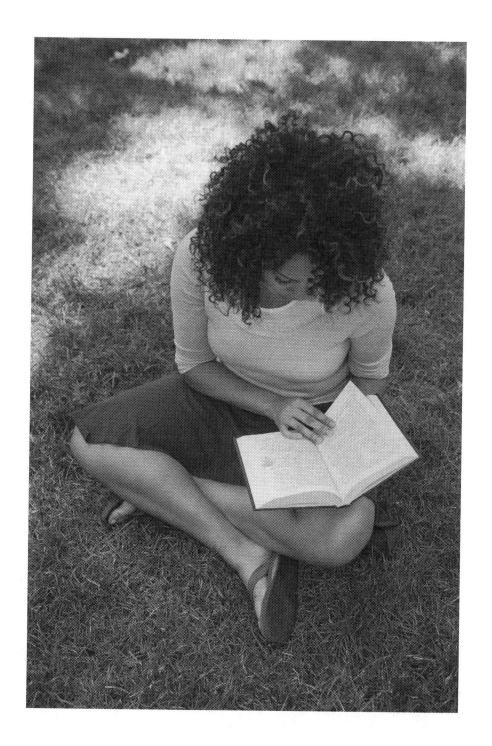

Sermon Notes

There are available now plenty of Prayer and Sermon Notes journals that can be found in many Christian book stores. Also, frequently, churches will have a place in the Sunday program made available for notes on the sermon. One of my Bible study teachers was the first to enlighten me as to the growth and focus that could take place through this note-taking practice. Using this approach helps you focus and remember the contents of the sermon long after Sunday. Remembering what was read and preached has been a problem for many others and me. This practice, I've found, also helps you stay awake during a lengthy, poorly prepared sermon, for example. Since I began the practice after his tip, I have never stopped.

My note taking has even encouraged others to do the same, including my husband. This same teacher also mentioned how it helped preachers stay sharp when they saw members of the congregation taking notes and especially when note takers would come up after service and talk about a particular point that stood out to them.

One company that makes personalized journals is Keeping the Special Alive Productions, www.ktsaproductions.com and ktsa1212@Yahoo.com. You may want to order from them a gift or a personal journal, made with your name or another's on it.

Following is a format you can use until you decide what you'd like to do or acquire or make your own sermon notebook.

Sermon Notes

Date_____   Speaker_____

Worship Place_____ City/State_____

Focus verses _____

_____

Title _____

Notes _____

_____

_____

_____

_____

_____

_____

_____

_____

_____

Action I Am Called to Do:

How I Can Apply This to My Life:_____

_____

Outreach: How I Am Inspired to Reach Out to Others:_____

_____

"You will seek me and find me when you seek me with all your heart." Jeremiah 29:13 (NIV) *"Faith without works is dead."* James 2:17 (NIV)

SECTION SEVEN
Growth Aides

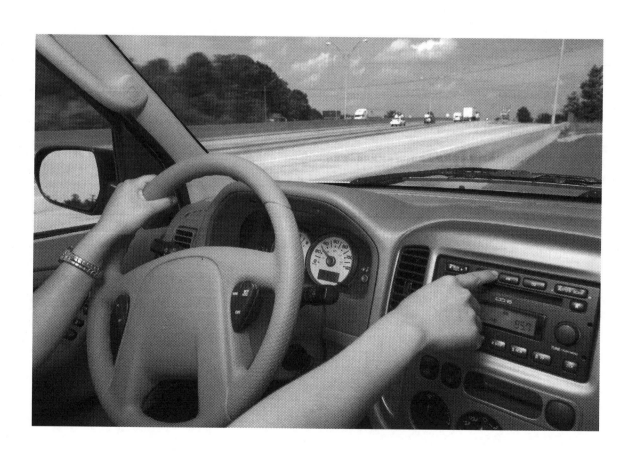

Growth Aides

Year: ___20_____

Books, tapes, CD's, Audiovisuals I have utilized for growth this year:

(See our web site: www.relationships-sweet.com or request our bibliographies for some suggestions)

_____ Month _____ _____
Resources/format _____

_____

_____

_____ Month _____ _____
Resources/format _____

_____

_____

_____ Month _____ _____
Resources/format _____

_____

_____

_____ Month _____ _____
Resources/format _____

_____

_____

_____ Month _____ _____

Resources/format _____

_____

_____

_____ Month _____ _____

Resources/format _____

_____

_____

_____ Month _____ _____

Resources/format _____

_____

_____

_____ Month _____ _____

Resources/format _____

_____

_____

_____ Month _____ _____

Resources/format _____

_____

_____

_____ Month _____ _____

Resources/format _____

_____

_____

"If the Lord delights in a man's way, he makes his steps firm: though he stumble, he will not fall, for the Lord upholds him with his hand." Psalms 37:23-24 (NIV)

Blessings!

If you have used this spiritual growth notebook for one year or even part of a year, you truly have invested wisely and should be seeing and benefiting from your growth. You are encouraged to try it again.

Carry on dear sisters and brothers. Your lover the great "Abba", Yahweh, Jehovah God and His son, Jesus the Christ, await to be even more intimate with you in this earthly, out of this world journey.

Enjoy the growing relationship and spreading the good news of the Kingdom! Life to the max! John 10:9-10

"I will never leave you nor forsake you." Hebrews 13:5b, Deuteronomy 31:8b NAB
"And behold, I am with you always, until the end of the age." Matthews 28: 20b NAB

Appendix

List of References

Bible References from:

The HOLY BIBLE, NEW INTERNATIONAL VERSION ®. Copyright © 1973, 1978, 1984 by International Bible Society.

The Message. Copyright © 1993, 1994, 1995, 1996, 2000, 2001, 2002. by NavPress Publishing Group.

The New American Bible for Catholics with Revised New Testament and Revised Book of Psalms © 1970, 1986, 1991 by the Confraternity of Christian Doctrine.

Revised Standard Version of the Bible © 1946, 1952, 1971, 1973.

Other References as they appear in the text:

Campus Crusade for Christ, (ministry and materials) 375 Highway 74 South, Suite A, Peachtree City, GA 30269. www.campuscrusade.org.

Our Daily Bread booklet, RBC Ministries, P.O. Box 2222, Grand Rapids, MI 49501-2222. www.rbc.org

1. Foster, Richard J. *Celebration of Discipline: The Path to Spiritual Growth.* Revised edition. New York: HarperCollins Publishers, © 1978.1988.

2. Bruce, F.F., general edition. *The International Bible Commentary with the New International Version.* Carmel, New York: Guideposts, © 1986.

Covey, Stephen R. *The 7 Habits of Highly Effective People: Powerful Lessons in Personal Change.* New York, New York: Simon & Schuster, © 1989.

Bass, Dorothy C. editor. *Practicing Our Faith: A Way of Life for a Searching People.* San Francisco, California: Jossey-Bass. © 1997.

Ortlund, Anne. *Disciplines of the Beautiful Woman, with built in study guide.* Waco, Texas: Word Book Publisher, © 1977, 1984.

Klingaman, Peter. *Finding Rest When the Work Is Never Done.* Colorado Springs, Colorado: Cook Communications Ministries, © 2000.

Shook, Kerry & Chris. *One Month to Live: Thirty Days to a No-Regrets Life.* Colorado Springs, Colorado: Waterbrook Press, © 2008.

Swindoll, Dr. Charles R. *Living Beyond A Life of Mediocrity.* Nashville, Tennessee: Thomas Nelson Publishers, © 1989.

Barnes, Emilie. *My Daily Planner.* Eugene, Oregon: Harvest House Publishers, © 1983.

Dillow, Linda. *Priority Planner.* Nashville, Tennessee: Thomas Nelson Publishers, © 1977.

LaHaye, Tim. *How to Study the Bible for Yourself.* Eugene, Oregon: Harvest House Publishers. © 1976.

Other Devotional Books and Spiritual Growth Enhancers

Casey, Michael. *Toward God: The Ancient Wisdom of Western Prayer.* Liguori, Missouri. Liguori/Triumph. ©1996.

Christenson, Evelyn. *Lord Change Me.* Wheaton, Illinois. SP Publications. © 1977.

Eastman, Dick. *The Hour That Changes the World: A Practical Plan for Personal Prayer.* Grand Rapids, Michigan: Baker Book House. © 1978.

Kelly, Thomas R. *A Testament of Devotion.* San Francisco, California: HarperCollins Publishers. © 1992.

Knight, Fr. David. *Reaching Jesus: Five Steps to a Fuller Life.* Cincinnati, Ohio. St. Anthony Messenger Press. © 1998. Small, brief, but very practical.

Munroe, Rev. Myles. *Rediscovering the Kingdom: Ancient Hope for our 21ˢᵗ Century World.* Shippensburg, Pennsylvania: Destiny Image Publishers. © 2004.

Price, Matthew. *123 Amazing Believers Every Christian Should Know.* Brentwood, Tennessee. Bell Rive Publishing. © 2004. Short biographical sketches.

Savard, Liberty S. *Shattering Your Strongholds: Freedom From Your Struggles.* South Plainfield, New Jersey: Bridge-Logos Publishers. © 1992. She has more great books.

Skoglund, Elizabeth R. *Found Faithful: The Timeless Stories of Charles Spurgeon, Amy Carmichael, C. S. Lewis, Ruth Bell Graham, and Others.* Grand Rapids, Michigan: Discovery House Publishers. © 2003. Down to earth, short, interesting glimpses of giants.

Tenney, Tommy. *Mary's Prayers and Martha's Recipes.* Shippensburg, Pennsylvania: Destiny Image Publishers. © 2002.

Teresa of Avila. *The Interior Castle.* Kieran Kavanaugh & Otilio Rodriguez, translators. New York, New York: Paulist Press. © 1979.

Besides checking Christian bookstores and on line bookstores like Christian Book Distributors for these, also *don't forget your local libraries* – public and university and "companions on the journey" like yourself who may also have them.

Title	_Order code_	_Price_
Being Single, Happy and A Chaste Christian Past 27	BSH	3.50
(A pamphlet) Durable cover		4.75
Engaged or Nearly Engaged, Landing or Loosing The Intended	ENE	3.50
(A pamphlet)		
Romantics/Aerobics Lovers, Exercise Procrastinators, Fountain Hunt	RAL	3.25

(A treasure hunt of beautiful fountains from the U.S. Capitol wading pool to 15th Street, NW and the Mall, *some hidden*.)

Monographs from Selectedly Singles Newsletter *(per pack of 3)*	SSM	4.75

(Great for singles groups' discussion, conferences, and reflection. Request a list with a stamped self addressed envelope, email us or see a sample on our site.)

Being a Prince and Princess of the Kingdom presented by Andrea Hughes	PPK	8.00

(Cassette Tape) one of several available. Request a list with a stamped self addressed envelope

The Singles Info Bookmark Collection: (Sheets of 3-6 bookmarks)	SIBC	3.00

9 Illusions Many Singles Have About Marriage, 7 Habits of Highly Effective Singles, 7 Dating Traps, 7 Reasons Why Cohabitation is Not Smart, 5 Quick Steps to Bypass Depression, For Relationship Fitness and Sexual Purity; *5 Traits of A Lasting Marriage, *How Again Can You Have A Lifelong Marriage? {*=<u>color</u> & blk. & white} **(Great for handouts, conferences, place settings, mailings and <u>your favorite single who hates to read)</u>**

What's So Great About Marriage? Lies, Myths and the Truth	WSG	**FREE**

A brochure (Send a stamped self-addressed envelope)

Some of the Resources Available
From EMBRACE - Singles Wholeness & Marriage Strengthening
edited by Andrea Hughes and friends

*Single Adult Ministry Training Manual 3rd edition.	SAM	24.00

(For Young Adult & Single Adult Ministry leaders. *Makes starting, developing, and leading the ministry and finding volunteers easy.*) This loose-leaf binder format is great for implementation

Order Form on next page

****

Visit our website: <u>www.abundantlylivingserv.com</u> or call us: 202-269-3449 for further order information.

Prices subject to change without notice.

Resources Order Form
All prices include shipping and handling

··

DATE OF ORDER _____/_____/_____ PLEASE PRINT ALL INFORMATION

CONTACT NAME: _____ ORGANIZATION _____

ADDRESS_____

CITY_____STATE_____ZIP _____ PHONE#_____(EVENING)

EMAIL_____

ITEMS by code: code_____   cost_____   code_____   cost_____
                     code_____   cost_____   code_____   cost_____
                     code_____   cost_____   code_____   cost_____

A sheet of Black & White bookmarks - $3.00   **Total of all items: $**_____
A sheet of Colorful bookmarks - $5.00   **Sales tax 5.75% $**_____
                                             Amount Enclosed $_____
                                             Grand Total $_____

Please make check or money order out to: ALS, except starred (*) item. *For starred item only, no tax is applied; make out checks to Embrace-SW & MS Inc..* Mail to: **Abundantly Living Services**, 1226 Jackson St. N.E., Washington DC 20017. For more information and updates on our activities call us at 202.269.3449

Resources Order Form
All prices include shipping and handling

··

DATE OF ORDER _____/_____/_____ PLEASE PRINT ALL INFORMATION

CONTACT NAME: _____ ORGANIZATION _____

ADDRESS_____

CITY_____STATE_____ZIP _____ PHONE#_____(EVENING)

EMAIL_____

ITEMS by code: code_____   cost_____   code_____   cost_____
                     code_____   cost_____   code_____   cost_____
                     code_____   cost_____   code_____   cost_____

A sheet of Black & White bookmarks - $3.00   **Total of all items: $**_____
A sheet of Colorful bookmarks - $5.00   **Sales tax 5.75% $**_____
                                             Amount Enclosed $_____
                                             Grand Total $_____

Please make check or money order out to: ALS, except starred (*) item. *For starred item only, no tax is applied; make out checks to Embrace-SW & MS Inc..* Mail to: **Abundantly Living Services**, 1226 Jackson St. N.E., Washington DC 20017. For more information and updates on our activities call us at 202.269.3449

ABOUT THE AUTHOR

Andrea Hughes is the founder and director of Abundantly Living Singles and Family Life Counseling and Consulting Services in Washington D.C. Born in Texas in a large action packed family and now serving in the Washington D.C. metro area with her husband. Andrea is a Licensed Professional singles and couples Counselor, Communications and Relationships Coach, Consultant to clergy in marriage and singles' ministry and trainer of singles and young adult lay ministers for over 15 years. She is a 2006 graduate of Shalem Institute of Spiritual Formation and has been offering Mornings and Days of Reflection since her singles ministry days over 20 years ago. Through leading multi-media relationship trainings, seminars, workshops, mornings of reflection, and mini-retreats, she has helped men and women, young and old, especially singles of color who have never married and couples of all ages find more purpose and focus to their lives plus live happier, healthier lives. Using her interactive style, participants always find they leave her workshops and enrichment series with helpful information, resources, insights and practical techniques not only they can use but to be shared with friends and acquaintances too. She is married to John Edward Hughes, a mental health interventionist and youth basketball coach.

Andrea is the author and producer of several other publications, some especially for singles, including the popular eleven year Christian newsletter *Selectedly Single, The Directory of Reasonably Priced Couples/Singles Retreat Facilities and Day of Reflection Sites- Metropolitan Washington Area and the Single/Young Adult Leaders Training Manual.* Andrea's articles have appeared in the *Washington Afro American Newspaper, Fortress Magazine* and the *Book Report.* She has appeared on Michael Lassiter's talk show "Matters of the Heart" on radio WOL 1340 AM and the "Community Notebook" on WCTN 950 AM and the Church of the Great Commission's TV broadcast "Save the Family" among others.

She is presently the Director of EMBRACE - Singles Wholeness and Marriage Strengthening Inc. as well as Abundantly Living Singles & Family Life Counseling & Consulting Services. Andrea is available for marriage enrichment, small groups, days of reflection and discernment and enrichment weekends and interactive, multimedia seminars and workshops using a blend of her librarian/media specialist, education, and counseling background.

Some of the workshops, classes and seminars she has presented and available to you are:

Smart Singles Marriage Readiness: Being Mate Worthy

Making Brilliant Date/Mate Choices

What the Church is Doing to Help Save Marriages & Families

Disciplines of the Beautiful Woman

Cohabiting Risks – What the Fellows Forgot to Tell You and Your Girlfriends

Sex Traps

Personal Renewal and Life Management

Oh No! I'm Involved with the Wrong Person Again

Grooming of the Prince & Princess

Breaking Personal Strongholds

For Days of Reflection and discernment, singles' mini-retreats, small focused Bible Study or singles growth groups focusing on becoming spiritually, emotionally and mentally whole and effective plus more, call, email or write: Andrea Hughes, Director, Abundantly Living Services, 1226 Jackson St. NE, Washington D.C. 20017, 202-269-3449, email address – princessayh@hotmail.com, web site: www.abundantlivingser. com.

For:

- singles and marriage ministry consultation,
- days of reflection and discernment,
- singles mini retreats,
- healthy relationships-building,
- relationship coaching,
- spiritual direction/companioning,
- couples communication training,
- singles and couples relationship resources,
- and speaking engagements,

contact:

Andrea Hughes, Director
**Abundantly Living Services & Embrace-Singles
Wholeness & Marriage Strengthening Inc.**
1226 Jackson Street NE
Washington DC 20017
www.abundantlylivingser.com
princessayh@yahoo.com
202-269-3449